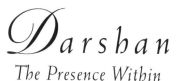
The Presence Within

Darshan
The Presence Within

by
Swami Vasudevananda

A SIDDHA YOGA PUBLICATION
PUBLISHED BY SYDA FOUNDATION

Front cover: *The sun illumines earth and sky, but the saint, kindling the fire of divine wisdom, lights up the heart. He is the true friend of man. He is the ātman [the Soul of the Universe].*
— Shrimad Bhagavatam

Lake Nityananda at sunset

Published by SYDA Foundation
371 Brickman Rd., P.O. Box 600
South Fallsburg, New York 12779, USA

Acknowledgments
The following people are gratefully acknowledged for their loving efforts: Cheryl Crawford for design and typesetting; Luis Barrios for the cover photograph; and Osnat Shurer, Sushila Traverse, and Valerie Sensabaugh for production. I also want to express my gratitude to the many people who so generously shared with me their experiences and revelations, some of which appear in this book.
— Swami Vasudevananda

Copyright © 1997 SYDA Foundation®. All rights reserved
Printed in the United States of America

97 98 99 00 01 02   5 4 3 2 1

No part of this book may be reproduced or transmitted in any form or by any means electronic or mechanical, including photocopy, recording, or any information storage and retrieval system, without permission in writing from SYDA Foundation, Permissions Department, 371 Brickman Rd., P.O. Box 600, South Fallsburg, NY 12779-0600, USA.

(Swami) MUKTANANDA, (Swami) CHIDVILASANANDA, GURUMAYI, SIDDHA YOGA, and SIDDHA MEDITATION are registered trademarks of SYDA Foundation®.

Library of Congress Catalog Card Number: 97-68976
ISBN 0-911307-57-5

Permissions appear on page 59.

Contents

Foreword
vii

Darshan: The Presence Within
1

Glossary
61

Suggestions for Further Reading
68

Foreword

This booklet is an introduction to one aspect of the mystical and sacred Siddha Yoga meditation tradition. Like the other booklets in the series, this text summarizes a wealth of teachings in a readily accessible form.

As you will soon discover, the teachings elucidated here are eminently practical and useful, addressing very real issues of daily life: how to become free from agitation and fear; how to move through life's constantly changing "ups and downs" with enthusiasm and courage rather than with dread and doubts; how to lead lives that benefit not just ourselves but others as well. These and other challenges find their highest resolution along the Siddha path.

The Siddha Yoga meditation teachings are based in the ancient mystical traditions of India. And they are very much alive, for they are imparted by the living master of the Siddha Yoga lineage, Swami Chidvilasananda. The extraordinary thing about such a master is her ability to awaken seekers to the inner experience of the Self through shaktipat initiation — the awakening of the inner meditative energy. Once this awakening occurs, our spiritual journey truly begins, guided very naturally and unerringly by the grace of the master. Swami Chidvilasananda is herself the lifelong disciple of the great Siddha Swami Muktananda, who in turn received the power and authority to bestow shaktipat initiation from his master, Bhagawan Nityananda of Ganeshpuri.

If you are new to the practice of Siddha Yoga meditation, these booklets will help you understand the basic truths and practices revealed and illumined by the Siddha Yoga masters. If you have been engaged in the practices for some time, you will find fresh inspiration for your spiritual journey. May these words — and the grace that inspires and enlivens them — lead you to the direct and blissful experience of your own inner Self.

Such a man is like a blazing fire,
 dispelling the gloom of darkness
 and burning the impurities
 of those about him. . . .
He is like a strong boat
 in which mortals may cross
 to immortality. . . .
The sun illumines earth and sky,
 but the saint,
 kindling the fire of divine wisdom,
 lights up the heart.
He is the true friend of man.
 He is the ātman
 [the Soul of the Universe].
 He is my very Self.

— SHRIMAD BHAGAVATAM

Darshan
The Presence Within

The longing to know God, the longing to live in the light of His love, exists in the heart of every human being. It is the longing of our soul to know its home, to rest in the fullness of what is our own true nature. Often we may live our lives not knowing what it is we're hungering for, and so we search in so many ways for nourishment, for something to fill us. Saints, great beings, exist in the world to awaken us to the experience that we already have within ourselves that which we are seeking everywhere. God is here with us. We can find Him *here*. We can know Him in our own lives and in our own hearts. Our hunger *can* be satisfied.

It is the work of a genuine spiritual master to awaken our inner vision, to reveal to us the divinity within our own being. A true Guru will never ask us to give away our power, but rather to fully discover it and to own it. Such a one ignites the flame of love for God within our hearts and also awakens the sacred energy each one of us carries within, for it is that love and that awakened inner power that will impel our spiritual unfoldment, wherever we may be in the world.

In the spring of 1996, Gurumayi Chidvilasananda paid a visit to the Siddha Yoga meditation center in Madrid, Spain. One of the people who came that day was a man from the Indian Embassy in Madrid.

I'd been speaking with him before the program and afterward, as Gurumayi was leaving the hall, I went to speak with him again. But he could hardly talk. He was holding his hands to his chest, and swaying, and there were tears in his eyes. Finally he said, "I never knew this."

"Knew what?" I asked.

"I never knew such greatness — inside myself!" Then he said, "I think this must be what great people do. They make other people great like themselves."

Actually, it's not that the Guru makes us great as much as she reveals the greatness that has always been there. This is the work of a Siddha master and the purpose of having her darshan.

The Sanskrit word *darshana* literally means "the sight of." On one hand it refers to the act of coming into the presence of a holy being or a deity, beholding that form, filled with divinity, and thereby receiving grace. In India, after thousands of years of this tradition, people intuitively know the value of even a brief moment of darshan, and they will travel great distances and undergo hardships to be able to have that moment.

Another meaning of the word darshan is "the perception of the divine." This includes having the recognition of divinity *within oneself*. Being in the presence of a true Guru — darshan — grants us the darshan — the perception — of God within and without. Though God is present everywhere, though God is present within our own being, it is through the grace of a great being that we are granted the eyes to see Him.

This is why the sage Narada proclaims in an ancient scripture on devotion, the *Bhakti Sutras*, "The darshan of a great being is rare, difficult to attain, yet unfathomable in its effect."

When you read the poems of the realized masters and listen to their songs, again and again you find outpourings of gratitude to their own Guru, the one who awakened their souls and bathed their eyes in the light of grace.

Guru Nanak, the great Sikh master, put it this way:

Though He dwells in each of us as our own life, though He is as visible as the palm of your hand, the only person who finds Him is the one upon whom the master confers his grace. By the grace of my Guru, I found Him in myself, and then my thirst was quenched.

"My eyes are filled with light," sang Brahmananda, a nineteenth-century saint of Rajasthan. "Once I saw only darkness in every direction, but my Guru has applied a lotion to my eyes and opened a pure, clear vision."

A Russian woman, who in 1996 traveled three days by train to be with Gurumayi in Łódz, Poland, wrote much the same thing in her own words:

It was as though the dust of centuries disappeared and my being was lit up by the grace of God, the Truth. The dust had covered my eyes, but the grace of the Guru took it away and changed my vision, made my vision sharper. Her love entered me. She entered my heart. Be joyful for everything.

Darshan of the Guru occurs in numerous ways. For many people throughout the world, the simple remembrance of the Guru draws the experience of her presence and guidance. There are others who may never have met the Guru in person but who receive her darshan through dreams and meditations, or as they contemplate her teachings or repeat the mantra she has imparted. And once our inner spiritual power, the *kundalinī shakti*, is awakened through the grace of the master, darshan becomes possible as an ongoing experience in the events of our lives, a continuous apprehending of the divine presence within ourselves and in the world through which we move. Swami Muktananda wrote:

*God and Guru give everything
but man does not know how to take.
Muktananda, what is the use of taking
just a little?*

The following pages depict some of the various ways in which the sublime experience of darshan takes place, so that we may open to it and allow it to guide and bless our lives.

*It was like a stream
    running into the dry bed
    of a lake,
        like rain
    pouring on plants
    parched to sticks.*

*It was like this world's pleasure
    and the way to the other,
                both
    walking towards me.*

*Seeing the feet of the master,
O lord white as jasmine,
    I was made
    worthwhile.*

— AKKAMAHADEVI

In the Presence of a Living Master

Whether we are conscious of it or not, we are continually sharing our inner state with the world in which we live. For instance, a truly compassionate person shares his or her good heart and, even without words, imparts to others the feeling that they are valued and accepted. An angry person, on the other hand, radiates anger. No matter how nice the words he may use or how much he may smile, what is communicated to us either subtly or overtly is anger. Such a person also projects that anger onto the world around him, constantly finding justification for his indignation or upset or rage. A fearful person sees the world filled with danger and shares his or her fear, and so on.

Swami Muktananda often quoted a teaching from the *Yoga Vāsishtha: yā drishti sā srishti*, "The world is as you see it." We are constantly projecting onto the world our own inner state of being, and it is that state which is communicated through our eyes, our voice, and the way we move through the world.

The spiritual master is one whose mind is merged in the Absolute, whose vision is filled with God's presence. No matter what roles we play, no matter how we have learned to see ourselves, she sees God in us, and this is the vision she shares. No matter if we have identified ourselves with limitation, or if we have created a facade to cover what we believe to be our imperfection, the master is able to constantly uplift us by seeing beyond these things to the purity at the core of our being.

Think what it means to come into the presence of someone who recognizes the purest, the truest part of you — the

light at the center of your being —
and who has the power to call that
forth. Someone who, through her teachings, her actions, her constant example,
says, "You can know this. You can live
fearlessly, knowing this. It is your birthright as a human being to know the
divinity living in your own heart." This
is the reason a Siddha Guru appears
among us: to share with us her vision,
her state, her ecstasy; to awaken that
state in us through the power of her
love; and to continually call forth the
greatness that each of us carries within
our own being.

When Gurumayi was in Poland in
the spring of 1996, I conducted a short
course inviting people to contemplate
and share their experiences. At one
point a man, perhaps in his early sixties,
stood up to speak. Looking into his eyes,
I sensed they had borne witness to all
the turbulence and tragedy that had
befallen Poland during his lifetime —

the concentration camps, the Russian occupation. Choosing his words very carefully and speaking simply and with great dignity, he said, "I thought I would never again in my life have anything to be enthused about. But I was wrong."

He went on to describe his experience of the previous evening. He had taken the weekend meditation Intensive with Gurumayi, which was held in the Opera House in the city of Łødz. After the Intensive, the singers from the Opera generously offered all the people who had been there with Gurumayi a splendid concert of operatic arias. As the man sat and listened to their beautiful music, his eyes were drawn to the chair that still remained at the center of the stage, the chair Gurumayi had occupied during the Intensive. In that moment, a scintillating point of blue light appeared before him and remained, steady and brilliant, throughout the performance. The man sat, transfixed, gazing upon that point of light, the light of his own transcendent inner Self. The pianist, the singers — everything faded into the background.

And as the man spoke of his experience and of the joy it had awakened in him, I saw that years of pain and bitter disappointment had also faded into the background in the steady presence of that light made visible to him through the grace of a master. "Today," he concluded, "I was looking at a photo of Gurumayi. She was smiling at me. And I know that what she has given me will always be with me now, in this new life." As the great poet-saint and mystic Kabir sang, "When you meet the true Guru, he will awaken your heart."

Students at the Siddha Yoga meditation ashrams or retreat sites might come upon Gurumayi not just in programs and Intensives but also as she passes through a lobby or visits the dining hall. She might be greeting a visitor, playing with the children, or walking in solitude by a lake or in a garden. You might even discover her standing beside you, chopping vegetables or washing dishes.

At such times, if your attention is directed even a little bit inward, toward your own heart, you discover that even in the most informal situations, the Guru is imparting her state and offering you gifts from within.

In the early 1970s, the first few Westerners had come to stay with Baba Muktananda in India at Gurudev Siddha Peeth, the mother ashram of Siddha Yoga meditation. In those days, Baba would spend hours with them in the courtyard, sometimes sitting silently but often speaking with them and answering their questions. There was one young American woman who noticed that Baba never spoke to her, although he seemed to speak readily to all the others. Days passed, and she grew more and more upset by this apparent exclusion. Finally one afternoon, after Baba had returned to his house and all the others had dispersed, this young woman was still sitting in the courtyard, staring at the patterns in the marble floor through tear-filled eyes, overwhelmed by feelings of rejection.

After some time, she heard the door to Baba's house open, and then she saw Baba's feet. He was standing right beside her, but she could not raise her head to look at him.

"Why are you crying?" Baba asked.

She did not answer.

"Is it because I talk to all the others and never talk to you?" She continued to stare at the floor.

"Listen," Baba said, "I'm *always* speaking to you. I'm speaking to you from within. But you never hear me."

The Guru is always looking for ways to uplift us and further our understanding and our progress along the spiritual path. Perhaps in the case of this young woman, what she needed far more than external signs of recognition from Baba was to learn to recognize and to honor her inner connection with the master. "All things are within you," Baba teaches us. "Receive from within." This is a wonderful teaching and, if we can assimilate it, we will find ourselves receiving nourishment and guidance from within even when we are away from the master's physical form.

So learn to come before the Guru as you might come before the ocean: You don't expect the ocean to say, "Oh hello, I'm so pleased to see you." You just take in the presence of the ocean, and you go away filled with that experience. You take the ocean with you.

Sometimes people who have a strong sense of the Guru accompanying them throughout their daily lives become confused when they arrive in the physical presence of the master. Seeing the

Guru smiling or speaking to someone else, they long for her to interact with them in the same way. Becoming distracted by externals, they let go of what they know in their own heart. And while it is a totally natural response to want to speak to the Guru or have her eyes fall upon you, when we seek her attention on the outside to the point of abandoning the inner focus, we overlook the great gifts that are constantly being offered to us from within, in secret and in silence.

Others, upon seeing Gurumayi in person, are disconcerted by her "human" aspect. Just recently I was speaking to a woman from the midwestern United States about her first Intensive. She was dismayed because, up to that point, she had been watching Gurumayi on video and thinking of her as some sort of "faraway deity" to whom she could pray. During the Intensive, the woman explained, Gurumayi seemed to be just like "a person," with a playful sense of humor and seemingly very human feelings. The woman was confused.

Put simply, the difficulty is not that the Guru is a human being; it is that we don't understand what a true human being is. It is the teaching and experience of the saints of many spiritual traditions that each human is inherently divine. This being the case, the true worship is to become great ourselves. And the role of the Guru is to constantly reveal to us that inherent greatness, that innate divinity, *our* divinity *as* human beings. She demonstrates what it means to be *fully* human. As Saint Clement of Alexandria said: "The word of God becomes a human being so that we may also learn from a human being how a human being becomes God."

*Behold, under the banyan are seated
  the aged disciples about their
  youthful teacher.
It is strange indeed: the teacher instructs
  them only through silence,
Which, in itself, is sufficient to scatter
  the disciples' doubts.*
— SHRI SHANKARACHARYA

In Silence

Baba Muktananda said that the true meaning of darshan is "to see a great being and become totally absorbed in his state for a while." And one of the most powerful practices of Siddha Yoga meditation is sitting quietly in the presence of the master, silently imbibing the master's state. Baba used to say that even though many people went to see his Guru, Bhagawan Nityananda, they would all become very quiet in his presence: "He didn't like people coming too close to him. He did not allow them to touch his body. Thousands of people would be sitting in front of him, but they had to be very quiet." As people kept watching him, Baba says, "they would feel him inside themselves and they would feel knowledge rising within."

It is said that when the eye touches the form of an enlightened master, we touch the *shakti*, the awakened power that flows through that form. Gazing upon the master, our being touches the master's state, opening us to the experience of our own divine nature. Baba wrote, "In Patanjali's *Yoga Sūtras*, there is a beautiful aphorism that describes this. It says, 'If you focus your mind on a being who has risen above attachment and aversion, then you also become free from attachment and aversion.' . . . When my Guru was alive, what I used to do was watch him. I watched him and watched him. By watching him I totally merged into him; I transcended the duality of the mind."

Late one afternoon a few years ago, a young woman finished her *gurusevā* — her selfless service — in the kitchen of Gurudev Siddha Peeth and came into the courtyard. Gurumayi was seated on her chair, silently repeating the mantra.

It was late afternoon. The courtyard was quiet except for the chirping of the sparrows who made their homes above the windows of the Temple and the light breeze that, every so often, would rustle the leaves of the mango trees and sound the tiny chimes that were hanging there.

The young woman's mind, however, was far from serene. She had come to the *gurukula*, the school of the Guru, after graduating from college and had spent several wonderful months there, embracing the practices and the ashram schedule. It had been a profound time of inner transformation for her, a time of revelation and self-discovery. But now the day was drawing near when she would return to her home in the United States, to start building her career and her life as an adult. As she thought about her new life, she was filled with trepidation. Where would she live? What kind of work would she find? All kinds of thoughts started going through her mind, and in her anxiety about the future she let go of her profound inner experience and got caught up in the whirlwind of her thoughts.

So this was her condition as she bowed and took a seat at the back of the courtyard. However, as she sat watching Gurumayi, she felt a wave of sweetness wash over her. The muscles of her abdomen relaxed, and she took a deep breath and closed her eyes — at which point, a voice inside of her said sweetly, "Could you just let go of a little bit of that stuff?" The young woman laughed to herself and found it an easy matter to let go of the thing she'd been fretting about just before entering the courtyard. And the moment she did, she perceived a soft light within herself. The inner voice continued: "Very good. Now, could you let go of a little bit *more* of that stuff?" She released another concern. In this way, the voice kept coaxing and cajoling her to keep letting go, and she kept following its direction until her mind was completely still and suffused with light.

The Temple bell rang, calling people to the evening chant, and the young woman opened her eyes to see Gurumayi rising from her seat and entering her house. Once again, she felt herself connected to the strong and blissful state that had been unfolding inside her during those months in the ashram. And she understood that her main work, when she returned home, was to keep remembering that inner light, to keep nurturing the inner *shakti* that would carry her to that experience again and again, through all the activities and events of her life. For it was from that place of connection with her own Self that she would receive inspiration and strength.

In the Temples of Bhagawan Nityananda and in the Samadhi Shrine of Baba Muktananda

The power of grace that flows through the form of a Siddha master does not depart when the physical body departs. Today, thousands of people who have the darshan of Bhagawan Nityananda's statue, or *mūrti*, in the Temples dedicated to him or who enter the Samadhi Shrine (the final resting place) of Baba Muktananda find the presence of these great beings fully alive there. These holy places are resonant with peace as well as spiritual power. There, we may find the apparent complexities of our lives dissolving into shimmering silence. Or we might discover the prayers and questions we've been holding in our hearts springing forth — along with their answers.

The *Shiva Sūtras* say, *dānam ātma-jñānam*, meaning that the gift that the master gives freely is knowledge of one's own higher Self. That supreme knowledge is constantly radiating from a true master, and it continues to radiate from the samadhi shrine of such a one or from the enlivened form shaped in his or her image.

Once a man was invited to assist in the *abhishek*, the ritual bathing of Bhagawan Nityananda's statue. As he carefully bathed and anointed the form of Bade Baba, he had the sensation that he was touching a conscious form of divinity, and he could feel powerful and blissful energy surging through his own body. Later, after the man had returned to his room and was washing his own face, he became aware that he was having the same experience as when bathing Bade Baba — as if he were touching a divine form of Consciousness. For weeks afterward, each time he bathed himself, he was drawn back to the experience of his own body as a living temple of God.

Again and again, people report occasions of Bhagawan Nityananda granting them guidance from within as they sit and rest in the immense peace that emanates from his form, just as it did when he inhabited a physical body. In the summer of 1994, for example, a young woman paid her first visit to the ashram in South Fallsburg. She was very new to Siddha Yoga meditation, had a restless mind, and experienced a lot of difficulty allowing herself to turn inside and discover her own inner being. Nonetheless, she was making a valiant effort.

One morning, she passed by the Temple and felt drawn to enter. No one else appeared to be there, only herself and the *mūrti* of Bhagawan Nityananda. She sat down, her eyes fixed on Bade Baba's kindly face. After a few moments, she began to hear what seemed to be a steady, rhythmic breathing. The sound was so assuring, so restful. She closed her eyes and started breathing along with that gentle, rhythmic reverberation. She had the feeling that Bade Baba was breathing with her to help her to meditate, and before long the sound of the breathing mingled with her own, carrying her into a vast, inner silence. More than an hour later, the young woman was still seated, deep in meditation. From that day on, the remembrance of this experience would guide her to a calm inner state whenever she sat for meditation.

For many people throughout the world, even the remembrance of Baba Muktananda's Samadhi Shrine in

Gurudev Siddha Peeth immediately draws them into a deep state of tranquility. It is difficult to describe the palpable love and the power that pulsate in this place where Baba's body rests, a place where you can almost hear the mantra *Om* rumbling like thunder. The air is always cool and sweet with the scent of flowers, and the mind becomes quiet there, held in scintillating purity, held in Baba's compassion. As Gurumayi has written, "You go to the Samadhi Shrine, and before you know it, your heart has dissolved from the sublime closeness you feel with Baba."

One morning several years ago, I was in a somewhat harried state, wondering how I was going to accomplish all the projects I had volunteered to complete in the time that they needed to be finished. However, by the time I reached the courtyard, I felt strongly pulled to Baba's Samadhi Shrine, and it occurred to me that, no matter how many tasks lay ahead of me, the most important thing I had to do in that moment was to give myself a little time to be with Baba. I went inside and knelt on the cool stone floor. After no more than a couple of seconds, I felt a powerful energy deep within — vast, compassionate, and invincible — sustaining me, *in* me. And with that experience came the inner command: "Stay here. Stay in this awareness. Don't run off after your mind. Stay here."

I walked out of the Samadhi Shrine just moments later, still immersed in that reality of being sustained from within. My mind was very clear, and over the next few days I watched myself moving through an intricate dance of activity in which everything seemed to come together exquisitely.

It's been several years since I've visited Baba's Samadhi Shrine, but still the inner command arises again and again as I mentally take a step through the doorway to offer my gratitude and my love. "Stay here; stay in the moment, fully aware of the great power that has been awakened within you. Don't let your mind pull you into its dramas. Stay *here*." And this experience never fades, but rather continues to grow ever more strong and to guide me back again and again to my center and my strength.

The Guru is always one with the all-pervasive Consciousness with which his or her awareness has merged. The samadhi shrines and temples of such great beings continue to grant their darshan and their blessings long after their bodies have departed from this earth. The ashrams that have grown up around them also are suffused with their living presence. Moreover, Bhagawan Nityananda and Baba Muktananda continue to appear in the dreams and visions of people throughout the world, sometimes answering their prayers, sometimes giving them teachings, sometimes guiding them to Gurumayi, the living master. As Baba Muktananda, speaking of his Guru, said: "Shri Gurudev's mission did not end with his body. It is even stronger now and continues to increase steadily. His influence is ongoing and will never end. It is not limited by space and time. . . . His presence is immortal, full of Consciousness, and all-pervasive."

I love reading Baba Muktananda's books. . . . I turn to them again and again. They are my prāna, my life-force. His wisdom is my courage. His wisdom is my life. . . . The messages of great beings are timeless. Their messages are inspired by the infinite light of the Truth, and therefore they always hold something new for you.

— Swami Chidvilasananda

Through the Words of the Guru

The words of a spiritual master impart the state in which such a being lives. They carry us from the realm of scattered thoughts and concerns into their world — the place of clarity and light in which they dwell. These words purify our minds, our intellects, and our hearts so that we begin to fully grasp and experience the vision behind those words: the vision of God everywhere.

The Guru is fully present in his or her teachings. Contemplating the Guru's words, we learn to go beyond appearances and to connect with the wisdom that dwells in the heart. That wisdom is the wisdom of the sages, the wisdom that produced the scriptures, and it dwells within each one of us as the truth of our own being.

It is the master's will that each of us comes to know that knowledge that we carry inside — to have the darshan of that truth — so our lives may be guided by that wisdom. As the great thirteenth-century poet-saint Jnaneshwar Maharaj wrote:

If your heart, through merit, should be illumined even a little by such wisdom, then every fear of life in this world would be removed.

Of all the words imparted by the Guru, the most potent is the enlivened mantra. Just as a seed from a great tree contains within itself another great tree in potential form, so the mantra holds within its few syllables the full attainment of the master. As Baba Muktananda has said, "The Guru always lives in your heart in the form of the mantra. See him right there; that is the best way of maintaining contact with him."

In Oakland, California, a man who was seeing Gurumayi in person for the first time spoke of how he had already met her — on the inside — while chanting the mantra *Om Namah Shivāya* at an Intensive conducted by some of the Siddha Yoga swamis. He said that as he chanted, he experienced an opening inside and found himself in a place that was filled with light, a place of incredible peace.

After a moment, he noticed that Gurumayi was there also, in that space of light within him, and that she was repeating the mantra as well. And he instantly knew that he had entered his own heart — that place of light in which the Guru resides — and that the mantra would bring him there again and again.

Before the Seat of the Master

❦

*W*henever Gurumayi enters a hall during a program or Intensive, before she takes her place on the Guru's seat, she lowers her head. She is bowing to the power of grace that flows through the lineage of Siddha masters, represented by the chair on which the Guru sits. In the meditation halls of Siddha Yoga meditation ashrams and in many of the centers throughout the world, a special seat, designated as the Guru's chair, represents this same power of grace. And when seekers come before this seat, it is traditional for them to bow, or *pranām*, signifying that they, like Gurumayi, are acknowledging that divine power that sustains and uplifts their lives.

Bowing is an act of pure humility, yet

it should not be understood as an abject action. Many people like to think of the moment of bowing as the time when they place their head below their heart and, in so doing, surrender the understanding of the limited ego to the greater wisdom that the heart knows.

Among the most touching sights I've seen are those moments when I've observed Gurumayi bowing simply and with indescribable tenderness and love before Baba Muktananda's Samadhi Shrine or before the form of Bhagawan Nityananda in the Temple. In her book *Kindle My Heart*, Gurumayi narrates what it was like for her when, as a child, she first saw Baba Muktananda, the master from whom she received everything, bowing in the Temple before the statue of his Guru:

All this time I had known him as a great being, an exalted one. I feared him, I was in awe. When I saw him

I trembled. Now I saw him with his Guru! And I saw in him what I thought I was feeling about him.

I saw him becoming small and totally soft. And though I was a very little child, and had no idea of the Guru-disciple relationship or about merging with the Almighty, no idea at all, I saw in Baba such purity and such an incredible amount of love that I just cried and cried and cried.

Bowing before the Guru's seat or the Guru's form is also a way of honoring the compassionate will of God, in service to which the Siddha masters have given their lives. These great beings have offered themselves so completely to God's power of grace that it flows freely through them. When we bow, we are asking grace to enter us and to flow through us, as well. Countless experiences have been shared by seekers who, after a moment of bowing, walk away restored and newly inspired after a long day of work; or filled with serenity, having forgotten the concerns with which they approached the Guru's seat. Although the Guru may not be physically present, the experience is one of having come directly into the presence of the master.

Following darshan of the Guru's seat, it is good to take a moment or two to turn within and notice the effects of that act of worship. This practice, like each of the practices of Siddha Yoga meditation, has the power to bring about a subtle shift in our awareness, to elevate us to a higher state than that to which we are accustomed. If we don't allow time after each practice to take note of what is happening within ourselves, the mind can very quickly close itself back into its habitual perceptions.

I know a woman who says that often when she goes for darshan and bows, the moment her head touches the carpet she herself seems to become completely transparent. Her mind becomes still and empty of all thought for that moment. For some time she was inclined to think that nothing had happened. But when she began to take a little time to sit quietly after each darshan, she started noticing that profound yet subtle experiences were actually taking place within her being as a result of that brief moment before the Guru's seat.

If it is physically difficult for you to bow, or if you prefer not to, of course you can still come forward for darshan of the Guru's seat and experience the full benefit of this sublime practice. The important thing is to come with respect, understanding that the divinity you are honoring in this way is the same divinity that you carry within your own heart, and that you can come to know it in its fullness through the grace of the Guru.

Through the Awakened Inner Power

―❦―

The most sublime manner in which the Guru bestows grace is through shaktipat, the sacred initiation in which the Guru's spiritual energy, the *kundalinī shakti*, ignites the awakening of our own. Once this has occurred, the inner power that was fully present within us, yet dormant, begins to unfold and to guide our transformation. In time we may become aware that, no matter where we are in the world, whenever we follow the promptings of our own awakened inner power, we are intimately connected with the Guru. For the Guru's life is so completely given in service to this evolutionary energy that she has become one with it. As Baba Muktananda put it, "In meditation you will experience your own inner *shakti*.

So understand that that is me."

Lately, I've been finding myself having many memories of the very first days after I received shaktipat in a Siddha Yoga Meditation Intensive with Baba Muktananda in 1974. When I went back to my home in New Jersey, I didn't really foresee that I would be able to meditate on my own. And yet I began to notice that there were times in the day when I felt the *shakti* moving in my body so strongly and sweetly that it seemed to call me to come inside in the most inviting way. If I listened to that call, I would be drawn into a state of profound silence and peace. Often, even when thoughts continued to move through my mind, it was as if I were independent of them, like someone who has dived deep into the ocean and is no longer being tossed about by the waves on its surface.

Encouraged, I set aside a room in my house specifically for meditation. I remember that room so clearly, and the sycamore tree outside the window. I can still recall so many of the experiences that took place there during those first months. Sometimes there were lights, visions, revelations. Sometimes there were movements: my body would sway or even move into hatha yoga postures. Sometimes my breath would move rapidly in and out as the *prāna*, the life-force, found a natural balance. I learned that these were *kriyās*, movements of the *shakti*, and that they were always beneficial because the *shakti*, being my own awakened energy, knew exactly what blockages existed within me and just what to do to clear them.

I remember in a very early meditation having a vision of the inside of my being, as if it were an old mansion with many rooms, all dark and dusty. A dancing, swirling energy came rushing through, flinging open the doors, pulling back the curtains, letting in air and light. In each of these sealed-off rooms there were shadowy figures, like ghosts, involved in different emotional scenes of conflict, violence, and despair. As the light poured in on them, all these ghosts evaporated and disappeared. Later I read about the *sushumnā nādī*, and how all the past impressions of countless lives are embedded in this central channel in the subtle body. I deduced that Goddess Kundalini was showing me how She was moving through my body and expelling all these old impressions.

Sometimes during meditation my chin would drop onto my chest, and I would pass into a state that seemed like sleep. That happened a lot, and for a long time. Years later I heard Gurumayi say that sometimes, when that happens, a healing is taking place on a very deep level. And it was true that often when I opened my eyes after one of those meditations, my mind was so still.

Everything looked the way it does after the rain — clear and lucid.

In time I found my life becoming filled with inspiration and my understanding of who I was undergoing radical changes. That house in New Jersey had once been a place where I had known an unbearable loneliness I couldn't explain to anyone, and now it was becoming a place I loved coming home to. I was discovering the company of my own inner Self. My life was becoming alive in a way I'd never known. I knew for certain that all this had come from that first Intensive with Baba, and I palpably felt him with me as that awakened inner power.

Gurumayi has said, "If you learn how to pay attention to the awakened Kundalini, She continually guides you. She is a living torch that guides you on your path." What She guides us to is an awakened life.

Wherever he turns his gaze, I am there before him. Even when he is alone, I am present there.

In short, there is none but Me everywhere, just as a pot immersed in water has water both inside and outside.

So he is in Me, and I am both within him and without. This experience cannot be expressed in words.

— JNANESHWAR MAHARAJ

Ongoing Darshan

Once the *kundalinī shakti* has been awakened and we follow the path the Guru makes available to us, we come to discover that she is always with us. The Guru stays with us in the form of her teachings, in the form of the practices that she has enlivened for us, in the form of our own awakened inner power. Furthermore, as the experience of our own inner Self becomes more and more accessible to us, we begin to apprehend the presence of God and the love of the Guru in everything we see. A simple occurrence — seeing rain falling on a leaf or a red bird in the snow — becomes an emblem of God's presence, a moment of darshan. Even the most commonplace events of our lives become imbued with divinity and grant us teachings. And we also begin to experience darshan through the presence of others.

Not long ago I was speaking to a young Australian woman who had been practicing Siddha Yoga meditation for several years. She told me that she had recently traveled to Greece, the country where her parents had grown up, in order to obtain some legal documents. While she was there she visited the village where her father had spent his childhood, and discovered that there was an old woman there in her mid-eighties — her father's aunt — who was sick and dying. When the young woman went to meet her, the old woman looked at her with great love and said, "God has sent you to look after me. I took care of your grandfather. He died in my arms. And I will die in your arms. Stay here and look after me at the time of my death."

The young woman felt compelled to

do what the old woman was asking, at least while she was waiting for her documents. Her relatives were very happy to take her into their home, as they had been worried about how they could give enough care to the dying woman.

From the beginning, the young woman felt close to the old woman, whom she called "grandmother." The old woman told her stories about her life, and in particular about the boy who had grown up to be the young woman's father. "He was like good wine," she said, meaning the best of the vintage, the wine that is brought to the church to be offered for the sacrament. As the young woman heard the stories, she gained a new appreciation for her own father.

However, not everything was so pleasant. The villagers were very suspicious of this young foreigner. They felt she had come at the end of the old woman's life to take away the inheritance, and, as is sometimes the case in little villages, they spent a lot of time gossiping about her and watching her every move. Moreover, living in the little house and being constantly under scrutiny, with people often staring in through the windows, the young woman felt it was not possible for her to sit for meditation or to chant. No one, not even the grandmother, would have understood. Nor was there a Siddha Yoga meditation center anywhere nearby that she could go to, nor anyone she could speak with about the spiritual path that had given such sustenance to her life.

Weeks passed, the legal papers still were not forthcoming, and there were times when the young woman, under the strain of her isolation and the weight of the old woman's suffering, felt that Gurumayi and the teachings were very far away, like a dream she had once had that was no longer real for her. And she prayed intensely for a sign that she had not been abandoned.

Then, one morning as she was serving breakfast to the grandmother, she asked the old woman if she had had any dreams. "No," said the grandmother, "but there is a woman who comes every night and sits by my bed."

"What woman?"

"I don't know her," said the grandmother. "She's foreign and dark."

The young woman caught her breath and asked, "Can you describe her? What does she wear? What color is her hair?"

"Long robes, dark red. I can't see her hair. She wears something on her head."

Trying to control the tears that were coming to her eyes, the young woman asked, "What does she do? Does she say anything?"

"Nothing. She just sits. But I know she's good, so I don't throw her out."

The young woman went out to the garden and wept in gratitude, knowing now that Gurumayi had been present with her all the time, helping her care for the old woman. The young woman picked some red roses and placed them on the table near the grandmother's bedside, and from that time on she knew that she was very close to the Guru, and she was where she was *supposed* to be, offering her selfless service.

A few more weeks passed. Gradually the grandmother stopped needing pain medication. She stopped eating and took only spoonfuls of water. She became more and more peaceful and started drifting in and out of consciousness. One day she died, quietly and serenely, as the young woman held her in her arms.

At the funeral, the village priest spoke. He told all the people: "This young woman was much maligned. People said many unkind things about her. But she was a great help, and she has paid a debt on behalf of her family."

At the close of the final public program of her visit to Melbourne, Australia, in the spring of 1997, Gurumayi said:

I will see you in different ways — through your dreams, through your thoughts, through your friends, through your family members. When someone says something, you will say, "Yes, this is the guidance I was looking for." You will know you are receiving guidance from the inner shakti. So, in the form of the inner shakti, we will meet one another all the time — sometimes in person, sometimes in other ways. We will be together when you see the moon, when the wind blows, when you drink a glass of water, when you go to sleep, when you chant, when you help another person, when you wish something good for somebody else, when you take care of your child, when you give love to your spouse, when you go somewhere, when you do not go anywhere. During all these times, we will be together.

On the path of Siddha Yoga meditation, the Guru is constantly seeking ways to make her darshan available to seekers. We're provided with books, photos, audiotapes, and videos. In addition, there are Siddha Yoga meditation centers and ashrams throughout the world where we can experience the Guru's presence through programs, courses, and Intensives, and through the company of other spiritual seekers. All these forms of darshan are there to gladden our hearts and support our lives as we walk the spiritual path.

Moreover, in time we come to discover the priceless darshan of our own inner Self. We become aware of how our own great hearts have become accessible to us through the grace of the master — one whose work in this world is to awaken hearts. Then we move through our lives in ever-increasing contact with the great resources we carry within ourselves, divine treasures that we can share with the world. With vision purified by the practices that the master gives and the unfolding of our inner power, we are more and more able to have the darshan — the apprehension of the divine — in everything we see. And we also know, with growing certainty, that wherever we may be, we have the Guru with us. For the one who awakens our heart also shows us how to come back to it again and again.

As Gurumayi has said: "The moment you enter your heart, darshan is possible."

―――― ❧ ――――

Swami Vasudevananda was a professor of theater arts at New York University when he first met Swami Muktananda in 1974. Six years later, he took the formal vows of monkhood. Since that time, Swamiji has traveled and taught extensively — on tour with Baba and Gurumayi and at ashrams and centers throughout the world. He currently offers his selfless service helping to train Siddha Yoga meditation speakers and teachers.

Sources

We gratefully acknowledge the following sources of quotes used in this book:

Swami Prabhavananda, translator, *Srīmad Bhāgavatam: The Wisdom of God* (Madras: Sri Ramakrishna Math, 1978).

A. K. Ramanujan, translator, *Speaking of Śiva* (London: Penguin Books Ltd., 1973). Reprinted by permission.

Swami Nikhilananda, *Self Knowledge: An English Translation of Sankarācārya's Ātmabodha* (Madras: Sri Ramakrishna Math, 1983).

Swami Kripananda, *Jnaneshwar's Gita: A Rendering of the Jnaneshwari* (Albany: State University of New York Press, 1989). Reprinted by permission.

Guide to Sanskrit Pronunciation

―❦―

Vowels

Sanskrit vowels are categorized as either long or short. The long vowels are marked with a bar above the letter and are pronounced twice as long as the short vowels. The vowels *e* and *o* are always pronounced as long vowels.

Short:
a as in c*u*p
i as in g*i*ve
u as in f*u*ll

Long:
ā as in c*a*lm
e as in s*a*ve
ī as in s*ee*n
o as in kn*o*w
ū as in sch*oo*l

Consonants

The main differences between Sanskrit and English pronunciation of consonants is in the aspirated and retroflexive letters. The aspirated letters have a definite *h* sound. The retroflexes are pronounced with the tip of the tongue touching the hard palate; *ṭ*, for instance is pronounced as in *a*n*t*. The following list covers variations of pronunciation for the other Sanskrit consonants found in the glossary entries.

c as in *ch*urch   *ḥ* is a strong aspiration
ṃ is a strong nasal   *ñ* as in ca*ny*on
ś is pronounced as *sh* with the tongue touching the soft palate
ṣ is pronounced as *sh* with the tongue touching the hard palate
s is pronounced as in hi*s*tory

For a detailed pronunciation guide, see
The Nectar of Chanting, published by SYDA Foundation.

Glossary

ABSOLUTE
The highest Reality; supreme Consciousness; the pure, untainted, changeless Truth.

AKKAMAHADEVI
An ecstatic, twelfth-century poet-saint of South India. Her devotional poems were often addressed to Lord Shiva as "The Beautiful Lord White as Jasmine."

ASHRAM [*āśrama*]
(*lit.*, without fatigue) The dwelling place of a Guru or saint; a monastic retreat site where seekers engage in spiritual practices and study the sacred teachings of yoga.

BHAKTI SUTRAS [*bhaktisūtra*]
The classic scripture on devotion to God, composed by the sage Narada.

BRAHMANANDA
A nineteenth-century saint who was a devout worshiper at the only temple in India dedicated to Brahma. A great poet and yogi, he expressed his learning and wisdom in the form of ecstatic devotional songs.

CHIDVILASANANDA, SWAMI
(*lit.*, the bliss of the play of Consciousness) The spiritual head of the path of Siddha Yoga meditation. A disciple of Swami Muktananda since

early childhood, she took the formal vows of monkhood in May 1982. Shortly before his death in October 1982, Swami Muktananda bequeathed to her the power and the authority of the Siddha Yoga lineage.

CONSCIOUSNESS
The intelligent, supremely independent, divine energy that creates, pervades, and supports the entire universe.

GURU [*guru*]
(*lit.*, *gu*, darkness; *ru*, light) A spiritual master who has attained oneness with God and who is therefore able both to initiate seekers and to guide them on the spiritual path to liberation. A Guru is required to be learned in the scriptures and must belong to a lineage of masters. *See also* SHAKTIPAT; SIDDHA.

GURUDEV SIDDHA PEETH
(*lit.*, abode of the perfected beings) The mother ashram of Siddha Yoga meditation, located in Ganeshpuri, India. *See also* ASHRAM.

GURUMAYI
A term of respect and endearment often used in addressing Swami Chidvilasananda.

GURU NANAK
(1469-1538) Founder and first Guru of the Sikh religion. He lectured widely, spreading liberal religious and social doctrines which included opposition to the caste system and to the division between Hindus and Muslims.

JAPA MALA [*japa mala*]
A string of beads used to facilitate a state of concentration on the mantra.

JNANESHWAR MAHARAJ

(1275-1296) A great poet-saint of India whose *Jñāneshwarī* is a magnificent commentary in Marathi verse on the *Bhagavad Gītā*.

KABIR

(1440-1518) A great poet-saint and mystic who lived as a simple weaver in Benares. His poems describe the universality of the Self, the greatness of the Guru, and the nature of true spirituality. These verses are still studied and sung all over the world.

KRIYA [*kriyā*]

A physical, mental, or emotional movement initiated by the awakened *kundalinī* to prepare the body and nervous system for higher states of meditation.

KUNDALINI SHAKTI [*kuṇḍalinī śakti*]

(*lit.*, coiled one) The supreme power; the primordial energy that lies coiled at the base of the spine in every human being. Through the descent of grace (shaktipat), this extremely subtle force, also described as the supreme Goddess, is awakened and begins to travel upward through the *sushumnā nāḍī*, ultimately reaching the spiritual center in the crown of the head. There, the individual soul merges into the supreme Self. *See also* SHAKTIPAT; SIDDHA YOGA MEDITATION INTENSIVE.

MANTRA (*mantra*)

(*lit.*, sacred invocation) The names of God; sacred words or divine sounds invested with the power to protect, purify, and transform the individual who repeats them.

MUKTANANDA, SWAMI
(1908-1982) Swami Chidvilasananda's Guru, often referred to as Baba. This great Siddha master brought the powerful and rare initiation known as shaktipat to the West at the command of his own Guru, Bhagawan Nityananda.

MURTI [mūrti]
(*lit.*, embodiment; figure; image) A representation of God or a deity that has been sanctified by worship and enlivened by a special ceremony.

NARADA
A divine seer; author of the *Bhakti Sūtras*, the authoritative text on the path of devotion to God.

NITYANANDA, BHAGAWAN
(d. 1961) A great Siddha master and Swami Muktananda's Guru, also known as Bade Baba ("elder" Baba). Bhagawan Nityananda was a born Siddha, living his entire life in the highest state of consciousness. In both Gurudev Siddha Peeth in Ganeshpuri, India, and Shree Muktananda Ashram in South Fallsburg, New York, Swami Muktananda has dedicated a temple of meditation to honor him.

OM [*om*]
The primal sound from which the universe emanates; the inner essence of all mantras.

OM NAMAH SHIVAYA [*oṃ namaḥ śivāya*]
(*lit.*, Om, salutations to Shiva) One of the mantras of the Siddha Yoga lineage; known as the great redeeming mantra because of its power to grant both worldly fulfillment and spiritual realization.

SADGURU [sadguru]
The true Guru. *See also* GURU.

SAINT CLEMENT OF ALEXANDRIA
(150-215) Missionary, teacher, and theologian whose ideas on monasticism and economics were influential in the early Christian church.

SAMADHI SHRINE [samādhi]
Final resting place of a great yogi's body. Such shrines are places of worship, permeated with the saint's spiritual power.

SELF, THE
Divine Consciousness residing in the individual.

SHAKTI [śakti]
Spiritual energy; the creative force of the universe.

SHAKTIPAT [śaktipāta]
(*lit.*, descent of grace) Yogic initiation in which the Siddha Guru transmits his or her spiritual energy into the aspirant, thereby awakening the aspirant's dormant spiritual energy. *See also* GURU.

SHANKARACHARYA
(788-820) One of the most celebrated of the East's philosophers and sages. Shankaracharya traveled throughout India, teaching and writing; he also established ashrams in the four corners of that country.

SHIVA SUTRAS [śivasūtra]
A Sanskrit text revealed by Lord Shiva to the ninth-century sage Vasuguptacharya, it is the scriptural authority for the philosophical school known as Kashmir Shaivism.

SHRIMAD BHAGAVATAM [*śrīmad bhāgavatam*]
An ancient Indian scripture consisting of stories of the various incarnations of the Lord.

SIDDHA [*siddha*]
One who lives in the state of unity-consciousness; one whose experience of the supreme Self is uninterrupted and whose identification with the ego has been dissolved.

SIDDHA YOGA MEDITATION [*siddhayoga*]
A path to union of the individual and the divine that begins with shaktipat, the inner awakening by the grace of a Siddha Guru. Siddha Yoga meditation is the name Swami Muktananda gave to this path, which he first brought to the West in 1970; Swami Chidvilasananda is its living master. *See also* GURU; KUNDALINI; SHAKTIPAT.

SIDDHA YOGA MEDITATION INTENSIVE
The primary Siddha Yoga meditation program, designed by Swami Muktananda to give spiritual initiation through the awakening of the *kundalinī* energy. *See also* KUNDALINI; SHAKTIPAT.

SUSHUMNA NADI [*suṣumnānāḍī*]
The central and most important of all the subtle nerve channels in the human body, extending from the base of the spine to the crown of the head.

TEMPLE
Unless it is otherwise specified, "the Temple" refers to the Bhagawan Nityananda Temple in Shree Muktananda Ashram or in Gurudev Siddha Peeth.

YOGA SUTRAS [*yogasūtra*]
A basic scripture of the path of yoga, attributed to the fourth-century sage Patanjali. It takes a seeker through eight specific stages, culminating in the state of total absorption in God.

YOGA VASISHTHA [*yogavāsiṣṭha*]
A Sanskrit text, probably written in the twelfth century and ascribed to the sage Vasishtha. In it, Vasishtha answers Lord Rama's philosophical questions on life, death, and human suffering by teaching that the world is as you see it and that illusion ceases when the mind is stilled.

Suggestions for Further Reading

Inner Treasures
Swami Chidvilasananda

In this collection of inspiring talks, Gurumayi Chidvilasananda offers practical ways to cultivate the inner treasures of peace, joy, and love, which are our birthright.

Kindle My Heart
Swami Chidvilasananda

The first of Gurumayi's books, this is an introduction to the classic themes of the spiritual journey, arranged thematically. Chapters include such subjects as meditation, mantra, control of the senses, the Guru, the disciple, and the state of a great being.

From the Finite to the Infinite
Swami Muktananda

This compilation of questions and answers is drawn from Baba Muktananda's travels in the West. In it, he addresses all the issues a seeker might encounter on the spiritual path, from the earliest days until the culmination of the journey.

The Perfect Relationship
SWAMI MUKTANANDA

In this classic work, Baba Muktananda unravels the mystery of the sublime relationship between Guru and disciple.

Where Are You Going?
SWAMI MUKTANANDA

A comprehensive introduction to the teachings of Siddha Yoga meditation, this lively and anecdotal book explores the nature of the mind, the Self, and the inner power, as well as such subjects as mantra, meditation, and the Guru.

Jnaneshwar's Gita
SWAMI KRIPANANDA

In the thirteenth century, the great poet-saint Jnaneshwar Maharaj composed this exquisite commentary on the *Bhagavad Gītā*, the timeless Indian scripture in which Lord Krishna reveals the Truth to His disciple, Arjuna. As Swami Muktananda has said, "Jnaneshwar wrote his commentary not simply through the intellect, but in the complete freedom of divine inspiration. He has depicted the very heart of the Lord."

Darshan Magazine

The monthly magazine of Siddha Yoga meditation explores the vast realm of spiritual knowledge. Each issue contains the writings of Baba Muktananda and Gurumayi Chidvilasananda, the teachings of saints of many traditions, sacred poetry, and the experiences of modern-day seekers on the spiritual path.

You may learn more about the teachings and practices of Siddha Yoga meditation by contacting:

SYDA Foundation
P.O. Box 600, 371 Brickman Rd.
South Fallsburg, NY 12779-0600, USA
Tel: (914) 434-2000

or

Gurudev Siddha Peeth
P.O. Ganeshpuri, PIN 401 206
District Thana, Maharashtra, India

For further information on books in print by Swami Muktananda and Swami Chidvilasananda, and editions in translation, please contact:

Siddha Yoga Meditation Bookstore
P.O. Box 600, 371 Brickman Rd.
South Fallsburg, NY 12779-0600, USA
Tel: (914) 434-2000 ext. 1700

Call toll free from the United States and Canada:
888-422-3334

Fax toll free from the United States and Canada:
888-422-3339